Frequently Asked Questions

all about
Pycnogenol®

RICHARD A. PASSWATER, PH.D.

AVERY PUBLISHING GROUP
Garden City Park • New York

D0816152

The information contained in this book is based upon the research and personal and professional experiences of the author. They are not intended as a substitute for consulting with your physician or other health care provider. Any attempt to diagnose and treat an illness should be done under the direction of a health care professional.

The publisher does not advocate the use of any particular health care protocol, but believes the information in this book should be available to the public. The publisher and author are not responsible for any adverse effects or consequences resulting from the use of any of the suggestions, preparations, or procedures discussed in this book. Should the reader have any questions concerning the appropriateness of any procedure or preparation mentioned, the author and the publisher strongly suggest consulting a professional health care advisor.

Series Cover Designer: Eric Macaluso
Cover Image Courtesy of Henkel Corporation

Pycnogenol® is a registered trademark of Horphag Research, Ltd. Pycnogenol French maritime pine bark extract is protected by U.S. patent numbers 4,698,360 and 5,720,956.

ISBN: 0-89529-906-2

Printed in the United States of America

10   9   8   7   6   5   4   3   2

Contents

Introduction

If you could take a single natural product to improve your cardiovascular system and reduce your risk of heart disease, would you? If you could take a single natural product to reduce inflammation, which aggravates arthritis as well as many other conditions, would you? If you had a hyperactive child, and you could give him or her a single natural product that might lessen his or her symptoms, would you? Of course you would. Any reasonable person would.

The natural product that offers all of these benefits and more is an extract of French Maritime Pine trees. It's called Pycnogenol (pronounced pick-nah-jeh-nol), and a growing body of scientific research and physicians' experiences shows that it can have a profoundly important effect on health.

Pycnogenol works for a number of reasons. First, it's a natural complex of several antioxidants—that is, substances that protect your body from free radicals and the ravages of the aging process. Second, it contains many of the beneficial compounds found in fruits and vegetables, but it concentrates them so you benefit from higher potencies. Third, Pycnogenol bears some similarities to the many natural herbal remedies sold, but it has a long track record of exceptional safety.

Pycnogenol has several key actions when consumed:

• It protects against dangerous molecules known as free radicals, which speed up the aging process and set the stage for heart disease and cancer.
• It strengthens blood vessel walls and reduces edema.
• It improves circulation.
• It boosts immunity.
• It helps relax blood vessels, thereby lowering blood pressure.
• It reduces inflammation.
• It eases allergies.
• It can help many people, both children and adults, overcome attention deficit hyperactive disorder (ADHD, or hyperactivity).

In the first two chapters of *All About Pycnogenol*, I describe exactly what Pycnogenol is, how it is prepared, and a little about its history. I also provide an overview of its health benefits and explain why it does so many good things for health. You'll learn a lot of new, unfamiliar terms, but I will explain exactly what they mean. In subsequent chapters, I delve into the benefits of Pycnogenol in greater detail and its amazing benefits in circulatory disorders, inflammation, ADHD, and other conditions.

Pycnogenol is a unique supplement. Although many different companies sell Pycnogenol, it comes from only one source. The makers of some other products may claim similar benefits to Pycnogenol but, again, there is only one product—patent protected—that comes from French Maritime Pine trees.

Sit back for a few minutes and read all about Pycnogenol.

1.

An Overview of Pycnogenol

A book such as *All About Pycnogenol* often begs as many questions as it answers. What exactly is this oddly named supplement? What can it do for your health? How does it work? This chapter answers many of these questions and provides an overview of this remarkable supplement.

Q. What is Pycnogenol?

A. Pycnogenol is a dietary supplement—that is, a nutrient or group of nutrients that comes in tablets or capsules. It is a complex of several water-soluble, highly bioavailable, antioxidant nutrients extracted from a particular species of Maritime Pine tree found in southwestern France. Many of the nutrients in Pycnogenol are bioflavonoids, a beneficial group of compounds found in plants. Pycnogenol contains several classes of bioflavonoids, particularly procyanidins. Some of these bioflavonoids are very simple small molecules. Other bioflavonoids in Pycnogenol are composed of larger molecules. In addition, there are also several "organic acids," also called fruit acids, found in Pycnogenol. These are also natural antioxidants.

Q. What are bioflavonoids?

A. Bioflavonoids, often called flavonoids, are a class of thousands of beneficial compounds found in plants. The structures of these antioxidant compounds enables them to easily donate electrons to other molecules. This ability to donate electrons, a type of subatomic particle, is a characteristic of all antioxidants. There are thousands of bioflavonoids existing in nature. Scientists have identified over 4,000 of them, but they are sure that there are several thousand more yet to be identified.

Flavonoids are found in fruits, vegetables, nuts, seeds, grains, cacao, and in beverages such as tea and wine. Many flavonoids are pigments that provide several fruits with their blue and purple colors, and some of the reds and emerald green.

In addition to their antioxidant properties, bioflavonoids have a host of other beneficial effects in the body. Studies have shown that bioflavonoids possess antiviral, anti-inflammatory, antihistamine, and even anticarcinogenic properties.

Q. What are procyanidins?

A. Procyanidins (or proanthocyanidins) are the class of bioflavonoids to which Pycnogenol belongs. About 250 procyanidins have been identified in nature. They were named so because of the blue hue they give to plants ("cyano-" means blue). There was a brief attempt to name these compounds pycnogenols, which means large molecules joined together from small molecules, but that usage was promptly discarded, and Pycnogenol is now used solely as a registered trademark to identify the product that is the complex of bioflavonoids from the French Maritime Pine trees.

Q. What are organic acids (fruit acids), and what is their role in Pycnogenol?

A. The array of organic acids in Pycnogenol is often overlooked by researchers who concentrate only on the procyanidins. These natural organic acids are potent antioxidants, but they also reduce the constriction of blood vessels and cramping of the uterus, which helps maintain normal circulation and reduces some of the discomfort associated with menstrual periods. They also stimulate the transportation of bile from the liver to the gall bladder, which helps promote digestion and the elimination of toxins. Caffeic and ferulic acids, two organic acids found in Pycnogenol, also help reduce the formation of undesirable nitrosamine compounds, which can cause cancer. Additionally, caffeic acid helps protect the liver from some toxic solvents and blocks the formation of undesirable leukotrienes, which are mediators of allergic reactions. Ferulic acid has significant anti-inflammatory action and improves capillary permeability. These actions are discussed in more detail later in this book.

The importance of the totality of the unique blend of procyanidins and organic acids has been demonstrated by studies in which Pycnogenol has been chemically divided into smaller portions. While one fraction shows superiority in one action or another, the benefits of the individual fractions never equals the benefits of the complete blend. The many diverse nutrients in Pycnogenol result in a synergy unmatched by any other known blend of nutrients. The smaller molecules provide antioxidant activity more quickly and can penetrate into smaller cellular compartments, the larger molecules provide a longer-lasting action as well as more diverse actions. Together, this blend provides actions not demonstrated by any other dietary supplement.

Q. Are the organic or fruit acids of Pycnogenol found in foods?

A. The organic acids found in Pycnogenol are also found in other foods, including various fruits, vegetables, nuts, seeds, and beans. However, nature does not combine these various fruit acids in the same plant in the same combination as in Pycnogenol, nor in combination with the same procyanidins.

Q. Where does Pycnogenol come from?

A. Pycnogenol is extracted from the bark of a species of pine tree that grows in the Landes Forest of southwestern France. The Maritime Pine from Landes de Gascogne is commonly called the French Maritime Pine tree. Its formal scientific name is the *Pinus pinaster Solander in Aiton*, which was described in the *First German Pharmacopeia of 1812*. However, it is also referred to in the scientific literature as Atlantic pine, *Pinus maritima*, Pin des Landes, *Pinus pinaster Sol.*, and *Pinus pinaster Aiton*. Regardless of the different names, it is the only species that grows in the 4,000-square-mile forest along the Bay of Biscay (Atlantic Ocean), situated between the vineyards of Bordeaux to the north and the Pyrenees Mountains to the south.

Although the bark is a by-product of the main lumber and resin industries, it is of special importance and receives special handling. The bark of the Maritime Pine is thick, dark reddish-brown, and deeply fissured. Its thickness protects the volatile bioflavonoids from evaporating before the nutrients are extracted. However, it is still important to extract the bioflavonoids from the bark within forty-eight hours of cutting down the trees for lumber. The extraction of Pycnogenol from the bark uses water and heat at the nearby Pycnogenol production facility.

Q. How does Pycnogenol work?

A. After seeing the long list of health benefits, you might wonder how could one supplement possibly do so much? Part of the answer is that Pycnogenol is not just one nutrient. Since it contains so many nutrients, it has several diverse actions. Some of the compounds act chiefly as antioxidants, others have antihistamine-like action, and others block the actions of undesirable compounds in the body.

Another part of the explanation is that some of the nutrients, such as the antioxidants, affect many body systems and thus are factors in preventing many diseases. Antioxidants are involved in reducing the risk of more than sixty diseases. The action of Pycnogenol in boosting the immune system explains how it increases protection against many infections.

Q. Is there research to prove Pycnogenol's health benefits?

A. Definitely. The discoverer of procyanidins, Jack Masquelier, Ph.D., conducted several laboratory studies that established Pycnogenol's health benefits. Several animal studies have also been conducted, followed by clinical studies conducted by the company that developed the commercial product. There are also several anecdotal reports stemming from thirty years of use in Europe and ten years of use in the United States. While these are important, what we will be concerned with in this book are the modern studies that have been done with Pycnogenol and published in the open scientific and medical literatures by American and European scientists. I'll describe many of these studies throughout this book.

2.

The History of Pycnogenol

Researchers now believe that they have traced the origin of Pycnogenol-like decoctions back to the fourteenth century. Much of the modern research on this antioxidant complex was sparked by accounts of how North American Indians used a Pycnogenol-like decoction to cure many of Jacques Cartier's explorers of deadly scurvy. In this section, we will recount the historical background and follow that lead to the forefront of modern science. Not only does Pycnogenol have a long and colorful history, it has proven its value over decades of commercial use with millions of consumers around the world. It has made a significant difference in the health of many thousands of people.

Q. How was Pycnogenol discovered by the Western world?

A. Before Pycnogenol was developed as a dietary supplement, there were reports throughout history of decoctions made from pine bark that healed various ailments. The earliest such reports have been traced back to about 1300. The report that sparked modern research was from Jacques Cartier's French expedition in 1535 to find a northwest passage to China. During the winter, the expedition became prisoners of the frozen Hudson Bay and had to stop at the North American Indian villages of Stadacona and Hochelaga. Because they had to spend the entire winter there, they exhausted their supply of fresh foods. The explorers soon developed scurvy, a severe deficiency of vitamin C. Scurvy had already killed twenty-five members of the expedition, and fifty more were seriously ill by the time Cartier befriended a local Native American, Chief Domagaia. The chief prepared a decoction from what was described as a conifer believed to have been pine, but could have been a tree commonly called Anneda or arbor vitae. The bark and needles were boiled to make a tea that was drunk several times a day. The men recovered within a week or two after beginning the treatment. The tea worked because the needles contained traces of vitamin C and the bark provided large quantities of bioflavonoids, which increase the bioavailability of vitamin C. Cartier wrote about all this in his *Voyages au Canada*, published in 1545.

Q. What is scurvy?

A. Scurvy is a disorder that results from a deficiency of vitamin C. It was common to early sailors who explored far from their home ports and, as a consequence, lacked diets rich in vitamin C. Scurvy develops when there is not enough vitamin C to produce adequate collagen—the protein essential for capillary and skin health. Without enough collagen to form the ground substance that fills the space between cells in the capillary walls, the capillaries leak so badly that they bleed. The symptoms of scurvy begin with muscle pains and weakness leading to total exhaustion with very little effort expended. The joints ache and even minor movement causes breathlessness. The skin becomes sallow and dusky. Deep depression soon sets in. The gums bleed profusely and the teeth fall out. In a matter of a few weeks after the first signs are apparent, the internal bleeding is so severe that it leads to lung and kidney failure and then death.

Q. Who figured out how Pycnogenol works?

A. Dr. Jacques (Jack) Masquelier of the University of Bordeaux in France, while he was a visiting professor at Quebec University in Canada, read of the story and became intrigued and wanted to find out why Pycnogenol cured the explorers. He began studying extracts of pine trees while in Quebec and continued his research when he returned to France with the unique species of Maritime Pine tree that grows in the Landes de Gascogne Forest, near Bordeaux.

His early research led him to report in 1966 that the vitamin C action of pine bark extracts was due to a bioflavonoid called *leucocyanidol*. He later named this compound "pycnogenol." In 1970, with the advent of better analytical instruments and funding from Horphag Research Ltd., he found that the extract was a defined mixture of organic acids and procyanidins. In 1984, G. Pirasteh, Ph.D., and Peter Rohdewald, Ph.D., identified and quantified most of the ingredients.

Q. How long has Pycnogenol been available as a dietary supplement?

A. Pycnogenol was first introduced in Europe in 1967 as an over-the-counter drug to treat circulation disorders due to problems of the blood vessels. It was first introduced as Flavan in France in 1967. Later it was also formulated in France as Resivit in 1973 and in Spain as Okavena in 1973. It is also known as Pygnoforton, Variflux, Venen, and Veden. As its popularity spread among health-care practitioners, it was given the more universal name Pycnogenol in 1987.

Pycnogenol was introduced as a dietary supplement in the United States in 1987. Since the research supporting the supplement was unknown in the United States, and there are strict regulations against making drug-like claims for dietary supplements, few learned about the health benefits of Pycnogenol. Also in 1987, Pycnogenol was granted a patent in the United States as a novel and powerful antioxidant and free-radical scavenger. At the beginning of the 1990s, the general population was beginning to learn of the health benefits of antioxidants. As more people learned of the antioxidant power of Pycnogenol, they also learned of its other health benefits. Slowly but surely, Pycnogenol developed a following, and today it is is one of the most popular dietary supplements sold in health foods and drug stores, as well as by multilevel marketers.

Q. Do doctors know about the many health benefits of Pycnogenol?

A. Surprisingly, many do. The holistic physicians (also referred to as orthomolecular or alternative medicine physicians) prefer to use safe, natural nutrients when possible because of the additional health benefits and lack of side effects. These physicians attend many nutritional seminars and study nutritional science publications and journals. A large percentage, if not most, of the holistic physicians recommend or prescribe Pycnogenol because of its proven benefits and their experience in their own practice.

Doctors normally learn of the benefits of drugs from pharmaceutical representatives called "detail" men or women. Although there are no "detail" sales persons to educate the conventional doctors about nutrients as there are for drugs, many conventional doctors have learned about the benefits of Pycnogenol from the success stories of their patients. However, the sad news is that not enough of the physicians have learned about Pycnogenol, and it may be another decade before this happens. Look at how long it took doctors to understand that vitamin E helps prevent heart disease. Now the majority of cardiologists take vitamin E themselves and recommend and prescribe it to their patients. In time, the majority of doctors may also use and recommend Pycnogenol.

Q. What research is being conducted on Pycnogenol?

A. Although research has been conducted on Pycnogenol since 1965, it is difficult to find the older studies in the scientific literature for two reasons: first the name "Pycnogenol" was not used until 1987, and second, most of the research was proprietary and not published in the open literature. However, several studies can be found. Extensive safety studies have been carried out under the direction of Dr. Peter Rohdewald of the University of Muenster in Germany. Past research on capillary health has been conducted by Dr. Miklos Gabor of the Szent-Gyorgyi Medical University in Hungary. Studies on Pycnogenol's protection of skin have been carried out by Dr. Antti Arstila of the University of Jyvaeskylae in Finland.

More recent research has centered on Pycnogenol's effects on heart disease, the immune system, attention deficit disorder, and Alzheimer's disease. Ronald Watson, Ph.D., of the University of Arizona, Tucson, has been researching Pycnogenol's action in boosting the immune system and protecting against heart disease. Dr. Lester Packer of the University of California, Berkeley, is studying how Pycnogenol works as an antioxidant and how it boosts the immune system. Dr. David White of the University of Nottingham in England has studied how Pycnogenol helps protect against heart disease. Dr. Schubert of the Salk Institute has studied how Pycnogenol helps protect against Alzheimer's disease. Drs. Stephen Tennebaum and Julie Paull, clinical psychologists in practice at The Attention Deficit Center in St. Louis are conducting a double-blind study with Pycnogenol and attention deficit hyperactive disorder (ADHD, or hyperactivity). As the number of scientific publications increase, there will be additional scientists eager to research the health benefits of Pycnogenol.

Q. Is Pycnogenol patented?

A. Yes, it is. There have been three American patents, two French patents, and a British patent issued for Pycnogenol. The first French patent was applied for in 1964 for the extraction of bio-flavonoids from pine bark. A use patent was applied for in France in 1965. The British patent was applied for in 1965. The first American patent was issued in 1969 and describes the use of Maritime Pine bark as a raw material for extracting medicine. A second patent was granted in 1987 for Pycnogenol's use as a powerful antioxidant free-radical scavenging actions. It was issued on October 6, 1987. The latest patent was issued on February 24, 1998. It is titled "Method of controlling the reactivity of human blood platelets by oral administration of the extract of the maritime pine (pycnogenol)" and lists Peter Rohdewald as the inventor and is assigned to Horphag Research Ltd.

Q. Is Pycnogenol trademarked?

A. Yes. The U.S. Patent and Trademark Office issued a trademark to Horphag Overseas Ltd. (a division of Horphag Research Ltd.) for the name "Pycnogenol" for dietary and nutritional supplements on May 11, 1993. An official logo depicting a pine tree encircled with the words "Pycnogenol French Maritime Pine extract" is often used on products and advertisements.

3.

Pycnogenol as an Immune Booster

Free radicals are harmful molecules that damage the body and lead to more than sixty diseases. They are involved in cardiovascular diseases and cancer, the leading causes of death among Americans. Free radicals also accelerate the aging process, and as a result are involved in decreasing our defenses against germs. Arthritis, Alzheimer's disease, and Parkinson's disease are also linked to free radicals, and studies indicate that antioxidants likely reduce the risk of these diseases. As a powerful antioxidant that also helps recharge other antioxidants, Pycnogenol helps protect us against the damage of free radicals very effectively and thus helps protect us from the more than sixty diseases associated with free radicals.

Q. What is an antioxidant?

A. Oxygen is a very reactive element, which is why it rusts iron, promotes combustion, and supports the life process. Iron and iron-containing objects that are left out in air (which contains oxygen) rust, or as chemists say, "oxidize." The process by which things react with oxygen is called *oxidation*. A substance that prevents or slows the oxidation process is called an *antioxidant*. Antioxidants also protect other substances, such as living tissue, against damage caused by oxygen.

In the body, it's important for oxygen to be channeled into the right places and kept away from other places. We don't want oxygen to react with vital cell components. This would damage them much like rust damages iron. In the body, unwanted oxidation of cell components can set the stage for aging, heart disease, cancer, and many other diseases. Antioxidants sacrifice themselves to protect vital components.

Q. What qualifies a nutrient to be called an antioxidant?

A. To qualify to be called an antioxidant, a few molecules must protect many, many other molecules. Our bodies make some antioxidants. However, we are dependent on the diet to supply many antioxidants. Important antioxidant nutrients include vitamins, minerals, amino acids, and coenzymes. Minerals are not direct antioxidants, but several minerals can become vital components of antioxidant enzymes made by the body. Such minerals include selenium, which is needed to make the antioxidant enzyme glutathionine peroxidase; iron, which is needed for catalase; and manganese, copper, and zinc, which are needed to make superoxide dismutase. Sulfur compounds, such as the sulfur-containing amino acids cysteine and methionine, help the body produce the most common antioxidant within cells, glutathionine. Antioxidant coenzymes, such as nicotinamide adenine dinucleotide (NADH), coenzyme Q_{10}, and alpha-lipoic acid, can be made in the body as well as obtained in the diet.

Q. How does Pycnogenol regenerate, or recycle, other antioxidants?

A. One of the reasons that antioxidants work together synergistically is that some antioxidants can regenerate other antioxidants. As an example, Pycnogenol can regenerate "used" or "spent" vitamin C, which in turn, can regenerate used vitamin E. This means that Pycnogenol makes a little vitamin C and vitamin E function for a long time in the body.

When vitamin E or vitamin C molecules come into contact with free radicals, they donate an electron to the free radical and make it a normal nonreactive molecule. This causes the vitamin E or vitamin C molecule to become a weak free radical. This weak free radical does no harm to the body, but since it has given up an electron itself, it can no longer stop free radical reactions by donating an electron. Thus, the vitamin E or vitamin C radical is useless and usually just breaks down and is eliminated from the body.

On the other hand, if the inactive vitamin C radical comes into contact with one of the bioflavonoids in Pycnogenol, it can be regenerated back into active vitamin C. Active vitamin C can also regenerate an inactive vitamin E radical back into active vitamin E. This effect of Pycnogenol is possible because the larger procyanidin molecules stabilize the lifetime of the inactive vitamin C radical so that it doesn't decompose and leave the body, but can last long enough to capture its missing electron from one of the many molecules in the procyanidin.

Q. What is a free radical?

A. You can think of free radicals as biological terrorists. Quite simply, they can be bad for your health. In chemistry, atoms that often are found grouped together can be called a "radical." This group or radical generally stays together during a chemical reaction and can be transferred from molecule to molecule.

Sometimes during very high energy chemical reactions, radicals can have an electron pulled away, causing the group to temporarily break free from the molecule. When this happens, it is called a "free radical." While this unstable, high-energy fragment is free, its energy forces attract an electron from other molecules. A free radical can pull an electron from most biological compounds, thus restoring its original electron content, but causing the other compound that has lost an electron to itself become a free radical. This free radical reaction can perpetuate until a key biological molecule becomes permanently damaged. Scientists have estimated that each cell in your body (and you have billions of cells) suffers 10,000 free radical "hits" each day. The amount of damage depends on how well the cell is protected by antioxidants. The higher your levels of antioxidants, the greater the amount of protection.

Q. What makes Pycnogenol different from other antioxidants?

A. First of all, Pycnogenol is much more than a powerful, multipurpose antioxidant. It also has strong anti-inflammatory, anti-allergy, and anticoagulant (anti-blood clotting) actions. All of these actions combine to give Pycnogenol unique and significant health benefits not known to be produced by any other antioxidant nutrient. As far as its antioxidant capabilities go, Pycnogenol is a very powerful antioxidant that is effective against many types of harmful free radicals.

Q. Is Pycnogenol the most powerful antioxidant nutrient?

A. It may be, according to the studies by Lester Packer, Ph.D., and his colleagues at the University of California, Berkeley. At least it's the most powerful antioxidant complex that has been widely studied under identical laboratory conditions and reported in the scientific literature.

When Pycnogenol was patented for its free-radical scavenging effect in 1987, it was described as being many times more powerful than vitamin E and vitamin C. This is certainly true under certain conditions. The specific laboratory test used to make the comparison (called the nitrobluetetrazolium, or NBT, test), however, is only one measure of a compound's antioxidant and free-radical scavenging capabilities. This test, which is done in a water-based system, is certainly not a fair one to use to compare Pycnogenol's antioxidant properties with vitamin E's, as vitamin E is not soluble in water to begin with. When comparing antioxidants, several factors must be looked at. One antioxidant may be better retained in one body organ or system or another. An antioxidant may be more efficient against one type of free radical or another. The only fair way to compare antioxidants is to compare their profiles of actions against various free radicals.

Pycnogenol has been rated the best of the many antioxidants that Dr. Packer compared for their effectiveness against several free radicals that are present in the body. In those systems in which Pycnogenol has an effect—which includes many systems important to health—he has found Pycnogenol to be the most effective of all nutrients he tested. The point is that there may not be just one antioxidant nutrient that is the best in all possible systems—but Pycnogenol appears to be the most powerful in the systems of major importance, and it definitely should be in everyone's defense against free radicals.

Q. Why is Pycnogenol such a powerful antioxidant?

A. An important reason why Pycnogenol is such a potent antioxidant is that it is a mixture of several types of antioxidants, so it distributes antioxidant nutrients widely throughout the body. The Pycnogenol complex of antioxidants provides compounds of varying sizes that can function effectively in different regions of the body over varying periods of time. The larger procyanidins are very effective in the bloodstream, whereas the smaller flavonoid molecules and organic acids can readily enter cell interiors.

In addition, the several types of antioxidant compounds in Pycnogenol make it a multipurpose antioxidant. The various nutrients in Pycnogenol have chemical structures that protect against different types of free radicals. Whereas a single antioxidant compound, such as vitamin E or vitamin C, is protective against a number of free radicals, a mixture of many different types of antioxidants protects against a greater number of types of free radicals.

Q. So, if Pycnogenol is so powerful, do we need other antioxidants?

A. The fact that Pycnogenol is a powerful and versatile antioxidant does not mean that it is the only antioxidant that you should take as a supplement. Many antioxidant nutrients work together as a team. Some simple antioxidants, such as vitamin C and vitamin E, are essential to life and must be part of the daily diet. Others, such as coenzyme Q_{10}, alpha-lipoic acid, and NADH are also involved in metabolism. These antioxidant nutrients have specific roles that are not replaced by other antioxidants. However, they can be readily consumed by free-radical reactions, and they are not abundant in the diet. Pycnogenol has sparing action on vitamin C and can regenerate used vitamin C into active vitamin C. Vitamin C can, in turn, recycle used vitamin E into active vitamin E. Vitamin E is fat-soluble and dwells in the body in fat-friendly areas, such as cell membranes and lipoproteins. Vitamin C and the bioflavonoids of Pycnogenol are water-soluble and dwell in the water-compatible areas such as the bloodstream and cell interiors. Thus, you should include as many types of antioxidant nutrients in your diet as possible. Pycnogenol should be included because it is a powerful antioxidant that has many additional health benefits.

Q. How does Pycnogenol boost immunity?

A. Dr. Ronald Watson of the University of Arizona, Tucson, specializes in studying the immune system and has conducted several studies with Pycnogenol and the immune system. In one study, Dr. Watson and his students found that Pycnogenol boosted the levels of immune components called cytokines (formerly called interleukins, or ILs), particularly IL-6 and IL-10. These cytokines decrease during HIV infection and lead to progressive defects in T-cells and B-cells, which are other important types of immune cells. All of these immune cells are also important in the body's resistance to cancer. In an experiment by Dr. Watson, Pycnogenol partially restored the decreased levels of IL-6 and IL-10 in laboratory animals infected with a retrovirus very similar to HIV. In addition, Pycnogenol greatly increased the activity of yet another type of immune cell, called natural killer cells, in both infected and uninfected animals.

Pycnogenol also strengthens immunity by protecting the existing immune components from their own chemicals. White blood cells use free radicals to destroy bacteria. When white blood cells overproduce free radicals, white blood cells start to commit suicide. Pycnogenol allows the bacteria to be killed while standing by to protect the white blood cells against any excess of free radicals.

Q. Does boosting the immune system mean fewer colds and flus?

A. Most likely. The clinical trials haven't been carried out yet, but boosting your immune system means that you will have increased resistance to all of the diseases caused by germs. Dr. Lester Packer suggests that, based on the study just discussed, Pycnogenol should be able to shorten the duration of colds and flus.

Q. How does Pycnogenol protect against cancer?

A. Many population studies have affirmed that diets rich in fruits and vegetables reduce the incidence of several cancers. Many scientists believe that the reason fruits and vegetables are so protective is that they are rich in antioxidants, especially vitamin C and bioflavonoids.

Pycnogenol protects against cancer in three ways: by destroying cancer-causing free radicals, by boosting your body's immune system so that any mutated cells can be destroyed before they become cancerous, and by reducing the tendency of cancer cells to stick together and adhere to other sites, in a process called metastasis. In addition, I believe that Pycnogenol will also be found to inhibit several tumor promoters. This effect has been demonstrated with other bioflavonoids and explains part of their protective actions against cancers. Dr. David White of the University of Nottingham in England has reported that Pycnogenol inhibits an enzyme (monooxygenase) from converting the precarcinogen in smoke, benzo[a]pyrene, into a carcinogen.

Free radicals damage the body's cell replicating system, which consists of deoxyribonucleic acid (DNA). DNA contains the templates to reproduce all of the cells in the body and is responsible for making "you." If this template becomes damaged by free radicals, the body may not be able to repair all of the damage, and the result is that when it makes a new cell, it may be a mutated cell, which can become benign (nonspreading) or malignant (cancerous) tumors.

Q. How might Pycnogenol reduce metastasis?

A. The process by which cancer cells travel through the bloodstream and attach to other organs (metastasis) requires that they attach to the tissue. This process requires molecules called cellular adhesion molecules (CAM). Pycnogenol reduces the availability of these CAM molecules. Without the adhesion molecules, the cancer cells are less likely to attach to other tissues and start the metastasis process, and are eventually destroyed. CAM molecules are also involved in allergic reactions, inflammation, and atherosclerosis, so reducing CAM molecule activity will reduce the risk of these diseases.

4.

Protecting the Heart and Circulation

There are several forms of heart disease, thus there are several causes. Most people think of a heart attack as the end result of heart disease, and most people associate cholesterol with heart disease. In this chapter, we explore the causes of heart disease and other circulatory disorders and discuss the cardiovascular benefits of Pycnogenol.

Q. What exactly is a heart attack, and what causes it?

A. Atherosclerosis, the medical term for narrowed arteries, does not by itself cause heart attacks. Narrowed arteries (blood vessels that carry blood from the heart) put the squeeze on blood platelet cells and damage them. Platelet cells are the cells that clump and clot in the blood. If you have a cut, they clot and keep you from bleeding to death. But in blood vessels, platelet aggregation leads to clots that interrupt the flow of blood. Clots can lodge in the narrowed arteries completely shutting off the flow of blood through that artery. When this happens, doctors call it a coronary thrombosis—a blood clot in a coronary artery. Hence, the expression that someone is having a "coronary."

When a blood clot shuts off the flow of blood in a coronary artery, the region of the heart fed by the artery is starved of oxygen and nutrients. The result is the death of these cells, which is called an infarct. This is the classic heart attack, called an acute myocardial (heart) infarction or AMI.

Q. What are some other common heart diseases?

A. Another common form of heart disease is heart failure, in which the heart is too weak to efficiently pump blood. Usually, the heart enlarges as it tries to compensate for the reduced output. Angina is the pain experienced in the heart when there is not enough blood reaching all parts of the heart during activity. High blood pressure (hypertension) affects arteries and is a risk factor in various forms of heart disease.

Q. How do cholesterol deposits form?

A. The process is very complicated, but it's important to remember that free radicals are involved and that Pycnogenol, as an antioxidant, is protective. Cholesterol is not soluble in blood, so it is carried in particles called lipoproteins. Two important lipoproteins are low-density lipoproteins (LDL) and high-density lipoproteins (HDL). The cholesterol carried by LDL, often called the "bad cholesterol," is carried to the cells from the liver. The cholesterol carried by HDL is often called the "good cholesterol" as it is being carried away from cells and back to the liver. Cholesterol deposits form only when LDL becomes damaged by oxidation—that is, by free radicals. It's then called "oxidized LDL." Oxidized LDL can infiltrate the artery wall and initiate a series of events that traps the cholesterol in the oxidized LDL. White blood cells, sensing that something is wrong, are attracted to the site and help form a lesion (cholesterol deposit).

Q. How does Pycnogenol protect against cholesterol deposits?

A. LDL is oxidized only when the amount of antioxidants is insufficient to protect the LDL against oxidation. The prime antioxidant that protects LDL is vitamin E. Pycnogenol can recycle vitamin C, which, in turn, can recycle vitamin E. Pycnogenol can also destroy the free radicals before they reach LDL to cause damage. The tendency to form oxidized LDL, and hence the cholesterol deposits (atherosclerosis), is dependent on two factors: the amount of LDL and the balance between antioxidants and free radicals. Both are important, but the antioxidant/free radical balance is the more important of the two.

It's also important to recognize that the so-called bad cholesterol, the LDL, is not bad unless it is deprived of antioxidants. LDL is needed to transport fat-soluble antioxidants (such as vitamin E) through the blood stream, which means it's essential for health. But like the rest of the body, LDL cholesterol also needs antioxidants to stay healthy.

Q. How does Pycnogenol protect against other causes of heart disease?

A. Cholesterol deposits by themselves don't cause a heart attack. They are a major contributing factor to forming the blood clot that causes the heart attack. As long as the blood can squeeze by the narrowing caused by the cholesterol deposits in good volume, the heart will receive sufficient oxygen and nutrients to keep the heart tissue alive.

A critical factor then is to maintain the proper "slipperiness" of the blood cells and prevent a blood clot from forming in the coronary arteries. Pycnogenol has a protective anti-aggregation (anti-clotting) effect on blood platelets. It is particularly effective against the damage to platelets from stress and smoking.

Pycnogenol's mild hypotensive (blood pressuring lowering) action helps maintain a normal blood pressure. Blood pressure is strongly influenced by nitric oxide levels in the blood, a compound that controls the relaxation of blood vessels and inhibits the angiotension converting enzyme (ACE), which raises blood pressure. Pycnogenol maintains adequate nitric oxide levels, controlling vasorelaxation and inhibits angiotensin converting enzyme (ACE), which promotes high blood pressure.

Many recent studies have also linked inflammation to heart disease. This inflammation, specifically of blood vessel walls, is likely related to the white blood cells drawn to oxidized LDL. Pycnogenol reduces inflammation.

Vitamin E is important to the heart and arteries in more ways than protecting LDL from oxidation. As an example, vitamin E is vital to maintaining a healthy lining of the arteries. Tears in the lining of arteries are another way in which deposits can form. Pycnogenol is a secondary factor in every way that vitamin E helps, as Pycnogenol regenerates vitamin C, which in turn, regenerates vitamin E. All of the antioxidants together form one terrific team to prevent heart disease.

Q. How does Pycnogenol protect us from stress?

A. When we are under stress, our adrenaline really flows. Unfortunately, adrenaline activates the blood platelets, so that they have a greater tendency to clump together and form a blood clot. While Pycnogenol can't make the cause of your stress go away, it can help by keeping your blood "slippery" (as an anticoagulant) to reduce the chances of heart attacks and strokes.

Q. How does Pycnogenol help keep the blood slippery and free flowing to prevent the clots that cause heart attacks?

A. Studies conducted by Dr. Peter Rohdewald in Germany and Dr. Ronald Watson in the United States show that Pycnogenol blocks the effect of the stress hormone adrenaline on blood platelets, thereby reducing the platelets' tendency to clump together to form blood clots. When a person is under stress, large amounts of adrenaline are released, which cause the blood platelets to clump together. Pycnogenol is particularly effective against increased platelet aggregation (stickiness and increased clotting tendency) caused by smoking.

Dr. Watson's research was presented at the American Society for Biochemistry and Molecular Biology annual meeting in May 1998 in Washington, D.C., and his research has since been submitted to a peer-reviewed scientific journal for publication.

In the study, a single dose of 100 mg of Pycnogenol protected subjects' platelets for 12 hours after ingestion, and a dose of 200 mg protected for up to two to three days. Regular daily doses at lower doses are expected to show the same benefit, and studies are planned to verify this.

This protective effect of Pycnogenol is achieved by blocking the hormonelike substance prostaglandin, which activates platelets so that they can form clumps when the body needs to stop bleeding. Pycnogenol inhibits platelet aggregation by inhibiting the enzymes thromboxane A2, 5-lipoxygenase, and other clotting compounds. Furthermore, this protection comes without an increased risk of prolonged bleeding times, or the side effects common to aspirin.

Q. Isn't this the same way that aspirin works to prevent heart attacks?

A. Not exactly—and the difference, though technical, is important. Pycnogenol inhibits the enzyme 5-lipoxygenase, whereas aspirin inhibits the enzyme cyclooxygenase.

Aspirin is widely prescribed by cardiologists to protect against heart attacks. The first studies showed that the proper dosage of aspirin can reduce the incidence of another heart attack in heart patients. Later studies showed that aspirin can also reduce the risk of having a first heart attack. So far, this sounds good, but unfortunately, many people develop serious problems with prolonged aspirin use. They can develop ulcerated linings of the gastrointestinal tract and an increased tendency to bleed. This can cause internal bleeding serious enough to result in death. Some people have been known to develop this condition suddenly and without warning. While aspirin therapy has benefit for many people, you should check with your doctor before taking it on a long-term basis.

On the other hand, Pycnogenol is safe and does not cause increased bleeding or the side effects of aspirin. In the studies by Drs. Rohdewald and Watson, it was found that 100 mg of Pycnogenol achieved the same desired effect on blood platelets in smokers as 500 mg of aspirin—and without the prolonged bleeding and other side effects of aspirin.

Q. How does Pycnogenol protect the linings of arteries?

A. Damage to the endothelium, or lining, of the heart and arteries contributes to the risk of heart disease. This damage can cause clots to form and allow cholesterol carriers to enter the artery walls. Researchers at Loma Linda University, California, studied the protective effect of Pycnogenol using endothelial artery cells. They found that Pycnogenol reduced the damage to endothelial cells caused by free radicals. They also noted that Pycnogenol increased the levels of other antioxidants in the cells due to its sparing and regeneration effects.

Q. How does Pycnogenol relax blood vessels to help prevent high blood pressure?

A. Pycnogenol does have a mild hypotensive (blood pressure lowering) effect that helps prevent high blood pressure. This effect is important, but it does not make Pycnogenol a hypotensive drug. There are two known reasons for this action. One mechanism involves the optimization of nitric oxide production in the blood vessels. Several researchers, including Dr. David Fitzpatrick of the University of South Florida and Dr. Lester Packer of the University of California, Berkeley, have conducted research on Pycnogenol and nitric oxide.

Nitric oxide has recently aroused much interest among scientists, though it was dismissed for decades as not being an important compound in the body— merely a waste product or inhaled air pollutant. Now, we understand that it has far-reaching effects throughout the body. Two enzyme systems control the production of nitric oxide. One enzyme system produces nitric oxide at a constant rate, while the other is activated by stress. Some nitric oxide is always needed, but too much can kill cells. Pycnogenol helps regulate nitric oxide levels in the body at optimal levels. It helps the body produce adequate levels of nitric oxide for necessary functions, while reducing the production of the enzyme that makes nitric oxide when too much nitric oxide is present.

Dr. Fitzpatrick conducted tests to determine the effect of Pycnogenol on portions of the aorta (the main artery of the heart). He found that it improved the production of nitric oxide in the endothelium, which in turn had a relaxing effect on the aorta. The results were published in the *Journal of Cardiovascular Pharmacology*.

Q. Doesn't Pycnogenol also lower high blood pressure by blocking an enzyme that increases blood pressure?

A. Yes, Pycnogenol blocks the action of angiotensin converting enzyme (ACE) in causing high blood pressure. In this way, Pycnogenol is similar to, but much safer than, common prescription drugs called "ACE inhibitors." ACE interferes with bradykinine, a compound that helps keep peripheral blood vessels properly dilated. Blocking this action leads towards a normalization of blood pressure without a danger of driving the blood pressure too low. It allows the bradykinine to act as it should, unencumbered by ACE.

Dr. Miklos Gabor and his colleagues at the Albert Szent-Györgyi Medical University in Szeged, Hungary, along with Dr. Peter Rohdewald of the University of Muenster, Germany, found that Pycnogenol has a dose-dependent action in blocking ACE from raising blood pressure. Based on their study, published in *Pharmaceutical and Pharmacological Letters*, the researchers described the hypotensive effect of Pycnogenol as "moderate" and people with normal or low blood pressure will not be affected, whereas those with high blood pressure due to too much ACE will benefit.

Q. Can Pycnogenol also reduce the inflammations that are now linked to heart disease?

A. Yes, it can. Evidence shows that chronic inflammation from ordinary bacterial infections significantly increase the incidence of heart disease. It may seem strange to find that ordinary infections, such as periodontal (gum) disease, are linked to heart disease, but inflammation activates white blood cells, which use free radicals to destroy bacteria and other "foreign" objects in the blood. Some of these free radicals leak out, oxidizing LDL and damaging the linings of arteries. Pycnogenol helps in a couple of ways. As an antioxidant, it neutralizes these free radicals. It also decreases the body's production of celllular adhesion molecules, which help bacteria stick to blood vessel walls.

Q. How does Pycnogenol improve circulation?

A. Pycnogenol helps maintain good circulation in several ways. One way is that Pycnogenol protects the endothelial cells that line the heart and blood vessels against free radicals. If they were damaged, the body would try to repair them, and this would result in scarring and lesions that reduce the flow of blood.

Pycnogenol also binds to collagen and elastin, which are important proteins in blood vessels and skin. While bound to these proteins, Pycnogenol blocks their degradation by certain enzymes. Pycnogenol also facilitates the production of "ground substance," an intercellular cement that can fill much of the space between cells in the blood vessels and control the amount of fluid and compounds that can slip through. This also gives the blood vessels strength.

Pycnogenol also protects the red blood cells so that they remain flexible and can squeeze through narrow capillaries. Pycnogenol helps maintain the efficiency of red blood cells in transporting oxygen.

Q. How does Pycnogenol strengthen tiny blood capillaries?

A. One of the earliest discoveries about Pycnogenol was its ability to strengthen capillaries, your body's tiniest blood vessels and the foundation of your entire cardiovascular system. Early research focused on the role of Pycnogenol as either an independent factor or a cofactor with vitamin C in the maintenance of capillary health. The earliest studies on the effect of Pycnogenol began in 1965 with Dr. Jack Masquelier at the University of Bordeaux in France. Later, Dr. Miklos Gabor of Albert Szent-Györgyi Medical University in Hungary conducted many studies over the years that demonstrate that Pycnogenol improves capillary permeability and decreases capillary leakage and microbleeding.

Capillaries are not designed to be sealed against leakage. These blood vessels are the interface between the blood stream and oxygen, nutrients, and waste products. Capillaries must be permeable enough to allow fluids to seep out of the capillaries, mix with the fluid that surrounds all of the cells, and then reenter the capillaries. If the capillaries are too permeable, too much fluid and protein seep out, resulting in edema (swelling), and even red blood cells may seep out causing bruising and red spots called petechiae.

Dr. Gabor measures the leakage of fluid through capillaries by using a device he invented called a petechiometer, which applies a vacuum over a small area of skin. The strength of the vacuum can be varied. The greater the vacuum required to produce petechiae, the less the permeability of the capillaries. Dr. Gabor and his colleagues have found that Pycnogenol improved capillary permeability within two hours and maintained it longer than eight hours. They have described their findings in the journals *Phlebologie* and *Scripta Phlebologica*.

5.

Effects on Allergies, Arthritis, and Other Disorders

The exciting news about the many roles of Pycnogenol in reducing the risk of the killer diseases, such as cancer and heart disease, has been uncovered fairly recently as researchers studied its antioxidant functions. However, decades before Pycnogenol's antioxidant roles were known, it was successfully used to control hay fever and other allergies. Its most popular use in Europe was for this reason. It has also been known for decades that Pycnogenol fights inflammation, although the reason wasn't clear until recently.

Q. What are allergies?

A. Allergies are hypersensitive reactions that occur when the body comes in contact with harmless substances that the body perceives as harmful. Substances that cause these reactions are termed allergens. When a hypersensitive person comes into contact with an allergen, the body releases histamine in an attempt to fight off the allergen. This release of histamine triggers the symptoms so common to allergies—inflammation, sneezing, runny nose, and itchy eyes.

Q. How does Pycnogenol ease the symptoms of allergies?

A. Pycnogenol blocks histamine release. Antihistamine drugs generally work by interfering with the attachment of histamine to cells after its been released. It's more efficient to prevent histamine release in the first place than to try to keep released histamine away from its receptors on target cells.

Pycnogenol also increases the uptake and reuptake of histamine into its storage granules, where it's out of the way and can't cause misery. A third important mechanism was reported by Dr. David White of the University of Nottingham in England. Dr. White has found that Pycnogenol blocks the action of an enzyme called histidine decarboxylase, which forms histamine from the amino acid histidine.

Pycnogenol is usually more efficient than antihistamines, without such side effects as drowsiness and dry mucous membranes. This may explain why Pycnogenol is the agent of choice for the treatment of allergies for many European health-care practitioners.

Q. Does Pycnogenol reduce inflammation?

A. Inflammation is characterized by swelling, pain, localized heat, and redness. It can occur due to irritation or injury. Fluid gets trapped in the spaces between cells in the injured tissue. This fluid most often is the result of leakage from capillaries, but it can also be produced directly in tissue via free radical reactions. Pycnogenol helps normalize capillary permeability to prevent the leakage of fluid that causes edema (swelling). It also helps by neutralizing free radicals that promote swelling and inflammation.

Q. So, can Pycnogenol reduce the inflammation of arthritis?

A. When people with arthritis take Pycnogenol for other disorders, they are often surprised to find that their arthritic aches and pains improve as well. This benefit should not be all that surprising because arthritis is a disease that involves free radicals and inflammation. Reducing free radicals eases the swelling associated with inflammation and improves the arthritic condition. A free radical called superoxide is involved in the inflammation of arthritis. This was demonstrated by the fact that injections of superoxide dismutase, an antioxidant that quenches the superoxide free radical, reduced the swelling and inflammation. Experiments by Dr. Lester Packer have shown that Pycnogenol also quenches superoxide free radicals.

Q. Does Pycnogenol help protect against Alzheimer's disease?

A. It's too early to tell, but laboratory studies are underway. One of the characteristics of Alzheimer's disease is the accumulation of beta-amyloid. Dr. R. Schubert and his colleagues at the Salk Institute of Biological Sciences, San Diego, have found that Pycnogenol prevents beta-amyloid (amyloid beta-protein) from accumulating in brain cells in laboratory experiments. They have also found that Pycnogenol protects brain cells from damage from glutamate. If you're interested in more details about these studies, and have a technical bent, the results are in the journal *Cell* (1994:77;817-827) and the *Proceedings of the National Academy of Science of the USA* (1992:89;8264-8268).

Q. Can Pycnogenol improve fertility?

A. Horse breeders swear by it, if that's any indication. It seems that antioxidants in general improve sperm motility and mobility. Especially useful are vitamin C, selenium, Pycnogenol, alpha-lipoic acid, and vitamin E. Dr. S. Roseff and colleagues at the West Essex Center for Advanced Reproductive Endocrinology in West Orange, New Jersey found that Pycnogenol improves baseline human sperm structure. They suggest that this 99-percent increase in structurally normal sperm may allow couples diagnosed with certain types of infertility to forgo *in vitro* fertilization in favor of less invasive and less expensive fertility-promoting procedures, such as intrauterine insemination.

6.

Effects on the Skin, Varicose Veins, and Bruises

In addition to the many health benefits of Pycnogenol, there are important "vanity" benefits as well. Pycnogenol is often called the "skin vitamin" or the "oral cosmetic" because it rebuilds skin tissues, making it more flexible and smoother, which makes skin appear younger and healthier. It can't undo deep wrinkles or repair permanent sun damage, but it can make skin healthier and smoother. In addition, Pycnogenol improves veins, repairing some varicose veins, and greatly reducing the occurrence of new varicose veins. Pycnogenol also protects against bruising and reduces the severity of minor injuries.

Q. How does Pycnogenol make skin younger looking?

A. As skin ages, it loses its flexibility. This is primarily due to the cumulative effect of sun exposure, which alters the skin structure and reduces the amount of skin protein produced. You can easily see this effect. When young skin is pinched and pulled up, it will spring back quickly. When older skin is similarly pinched, it returns to position very slowly. Try this on the back of the hands of people of various ages. How does your skin do?

Have you ever noticed that the skin on the back of the necks of farmers and fishermen is thick, leathery, and deeply wrinkled compared to the skin of office workers? You can also compare the apparent age of skin on different areas of your own body. We tend to think of the skin of our bodies as being the same age as our chronological age, but the fact is that some cells are much newer than others. Compare the smoothness of the skin on a sun-exposed area, such as the back of your neck, to the skin on a sun-protected area, such as your buttocks. The sun is what made the difference, by causing free radicals that fused molecules of the skin protein collagen together.

The proteins in young skin freely slide over each other and spring back to their normal length when stretched. As time goes by and exposure to the sun accumulates, the ultraviolet energy in sunlight interacts with fats in the skin to produce free radicals. These free radicals damage proteins in the skin and can link the proteins together. These damaged proteins do not easily slide over one another and do not recoil rapidly. How does Pycnogenol fit in? By neutralizing free radicals, Pycnogenol can lessen sun damage to skin.

Q. Can Pycnogenol help protect from sunburn as well as the long-term damage that ages skin?

A. To some extent it can. People who are well protected by antioxidants, including Pycnogenol, vitamin E, vitamin C, carotenoids, and selenium, do not burn as quickly in the sun. Sunburn is an inflammation resulting from the free-radicals produced by the effect of sunlight on fats in the skin. Free-radical damage can be limited by the scavenging effect of the antioxidants. Studies have shown that the time of exposure required for sunburn to develop can be increased with Pycnogenol, but Pycnogenol should not be your only protection from the sun. The use of sunblock, wearing a hat, and an awareness of exposure time are also important.

Q. Can Pycnogenol be used as an external sunscreen as well as an internal sunscreen?

A. Yes, it can. In experiments, Dr. Antti Arstila and his colleagues at the University of Jyvaeskylae, Finland, marked different areas of the forearm, applied different strengths of Pycnogenol to these areas, then exposed the forearm to sunlight. Pycnogenol protected the skin in a dose-related manner, meaning that higher concentrations were better than lower concentrations.

Q. How does Pycnogenol contribute to skin smoothness?

A. In addition to its protective benefits against free

radicals, which prevents skin damage, Pycnogenol binds to collagen, a major protein in skin, and protects it from various enzymes that break it down. This action reduces the thinning of skin that develops with aging. Pycnogenol helps the skin rebuild its thickness and elasticity. Skin fullness and elasticity are essential for skin smoothness.

Q. Can Pycnogenol cure psoriasis?

A. Psoriasis is characterized by capillary bleeding associated with increased capillary fragility. The capillary resistance of psoriatic patients is significantly lower than that of healthy persons. According to Dr. Miklos Gabor of the Albert Szent-Gyorgyi Medical University, Hungary, Pycnogenol tends to restore normal capillary resistance in psoriatic patients.

Although there are no clinical studies to verify this action, holistic physicians in Europe and in the United States have experienced good effects with Pycnogenol in psoriasis. Many have unexpectedly found that when Pycnogenol was given to patients for other disorders, the patients' psoriasis suddenly cleared up.

Q. Does Pycnogenol protect against varicose veins?

A. Dr. F. Feine-Haake of Horphag Research Ltd., studied the benefit of 30 mg of Pycnogenol given three times a day (a total of 90 mgs) on 100 persons having varicose veins. Eighty percent showed a clear improvement, and 90 percent of them found that their nocturnal leg cramps also disappeared. Pycnogenol helps keep all of the blood vessels healthy and reduces edema in the legs, which contributes to the development of varicose veins. Some of the first uses of Pycnogenol were for weak or poor functioning veins, restless legs, and edema.

Q. How does Pycnogenol prevent bruising and reduce the severity of minor injuries?

A. Pycnogenol helps maintain capillary strength and proper capillary permeability. A bruise is pooled blood beneath the surface of the skin. If the capillaries leak too much, fluid and proteins can leak through the capillaries into the neighboring cells, thereby altering the normal osmotic pressure. Eventually, even red blood cells can leak through and spontaneously cause a bruise without a direct injury to the capillaries. Pycnogenol restores proper permeability and reduces the incidence of spontaneous bruising. With stronger capillaries, it will take a more forceful injury to damage the veins and capillaries enough to allow microbleeding into the tissues.

7.

In the Treatment of Attention Deficit Hyperactivity Disorder (ADHD)

Attention deficit disorder (ADD) and attention deficit hyperactive disorder (ADHD) are a group of behavioral problems that used to be called hyperactivity. They involve impulsive behavior, the inability to keep focused on a task, and/or hyperactivity. I learned quite unexpectedly that Pycnogenol is helpful in the treatment of these disorders as well.

Q. How many people are affected by ADD and ADHD, and are they all children?

A. ADD and ADHD affect about 5 to 7 percent of the population. ADD and ADHD affects males about ten times more often than females. These conditions normally begin by four to seven years of age and seem to peak between eight and ten years of age. However, adolescents and adults also suffer from ADD and ADHD. From 30 to 70 percent of affected children are left untreated and grow to become adults with these disorders. ADD and ADHD rarely manifest themselves as adult-onset disorders. The physical hyperactivity lessens with age, but the adult still has marked attention problems and can be impulsive. Problems in the adolescent and adult occur predominantly as academic failure, low self-esteem, and difficulty learning appropriate social behavior. Often, those with ADD and ADHD have personality-trait disorders, antisocial behavior, short attention spans, and poor social skills, and are impulsive and restless.

Q. What is the cause of ADD?

A. The cause of ADD and ADHD is not known, but structural abnormalities have been ruled out. The leading suspect appears to be problems with neurotransmitters, possibly associated with decreased activity or stimulation in the upper brainstem and frontal midbrain. There is also suspicion that toxins, environmental problems, or neurologic immaturity could be causative factors.

Q. All kids seem a little hyperactive at one time or another. What are the official symptoms of ADD?

A. The American Psychiatric Association lists fourteen signs, of which at least eight must be present for a child to be officially classified as ADD. These fourteen signs are:

1. Often fidgeting with hands or feet, or squirming while seated.

2. Having difficulty remaining seated when required to do so.

3. Being easily distracted by extraneous stimuli.

4. Having difficulty awaiting turn in games or group activities.

5. Often blurting out answers before questions are completed.

6. Having difficulty in following instructions.

7. Having difficulty sustaining attention in tasks or play activities.

8. Often shifting from one uncompleted task to another.

9. Having difficulty playing quietly.

10. Often talking excessively.

11. Often interrupting or intruding on others.

12. Often not listening to what is being said.

13. Often forgetting things necessary for tasks or activities.

14. Often engaging in physically dangerous activities without considering possible consequences.

Q. What is the conventional treatment for ADD?

A. The conventional treatment is with central nervous system stimulants, such as amphetamines. Stimulants seem to have a calming effect on children. Ritalin (methylphenidate hydrochloride) is widely prescribed, and some people have estimated that 5 to 10 percent of our youngsters go to school on this prescription drug. According to the *Merck Manual*, common side effects of Ritalin are sleep disturbances, depression, headache, stomachache, suppressed appetite, elevated blood pressure, decreased learning, behavioral changes, and reduction of growth.

Q. How does Pycnogenol help those with ADD?

A. One way is that the antioxidant effect of Pycnogenol keeps neurotransmitters functioning longer. Pycnogenol also improves circulation, including microcirculation in the brain. However, I suspect that the effect of Pycnogenol is more complex than this. It will take more research to uncover exactly how Pycnogenol functions to help those with ADD and to improve cognitive function in general.

Q. How was the benefit of Pycnogenol to those with ADD discovered?

A. I'll take credit for being the first to report this at a scientific meeting, but the discovery has been made unexpectedly by many individuals. A common example is that persons taking Pycnogenol for their hay fever found that their ADD symptoms decreased in a week or two. Through the years, because I was the author of two other books on Pycnogenol, I have received hundreds of letters reporting this.

I surveyed the case histories and recent experience of several patients and found that Pycnogenol had helped all of the patients who tried it. I reported this small study at The Second International Pycnogenol Symposium in May 1995 in Biarritz, France. In August 1995, I received a letter from psychologist Julie Paull, Ph.D., who confirmed that Pycnogenol had also helped her immensely. Dr.

Paull and her colleague Stephen Tennebaum, Ph.D., are conducting a formal clinical study on Pycnogenol and ADD. At this early stage, they can only report that it is obvious that Pycnogenol helps to increase their attention and improve their focus, and may be decreasing their emotional reactivity.

8.

How to Use Pycnogenol

If you now believe that Pycnogenol may help you, you'll probably want some information on how to take it. This final chapter answers these practical, everyday questions. Select a brand that you trust, determine the concentration suited for your purposes, and double-check to see if the label carries the Pycnogenol trademark or patent number, or mentions that it was produced by Horphag Research. If none of these notations appear on the label, you have an imitation, not Pycnogenol.

Q. How much Pycnogenol do I need?

A. This depends on why you wish to take

Pycnogenol. If you just want to improve the synergistic effect of your nutritional antioxidants, you need only 20 to 25 mg of Pycnogenol a day. If you are seeking to optimize your antioxidant defenses, you may wish to take 50 to 100 mg a day. If you wish to treat a condition, such as hay fever or ADD, protect your blood platelets from stress or smoke, or reduce pain or swelling, then you may need to take one-half to one mg for every pound of your body weight. As the condition improves, you may be able to start cutting this back to the 50 to 100 mg per day range.

Q. Is it better to take Pycnogenol on an empty stomach or with meals?

A. Taking Pycnogenol with meals or on an empty stomach does not affect absorption, and Pycnogenol doesn't produce any digestive disturbances, so it really doesn't matter when you take it. However, most people find that taking supplements with meals is easier, more convenient, and gentler on the system. Bioflavonoids, such as Pycnogenol, improve the absorption of vitamin C, so it is wise to take Pycnogenol with your other supplements, and it is probably more convenient to take Pycnogenol at the same time you take your other supplements.

Q. Is it better to take Pycnogenol in the morning or at night?

A. As with vitamin C and other water-soluble nutrients, Pycnogenol is most effective when taken in divided dosages spread out over two or three times a day. This maintains a constant level of Pycnogenol in the blood. However, there is no reason that your daily amount of Pycnogenol cannot be taken all at once, at any time.

Q. Is Pycnogenol safe to take?

A. Yes, it is. Millions of users regularly take Pycnogenol as a dietary supplement and to improve many health conditions. Pycnogenol has been in wide usage since the late 1960s with no reported adverse health effects. It has been studied by toxicologists who have concluded that Pycnogenol is as safe as vitamin C, with less side effects.

Pycnogenol is nontoxic, nonmutagenic (doesn't cause mutations in DNA), noncarcinogenic (doesn't cause cancer), and will not cause birth defects in the unborn child of a woman taking it. Dr. Peter Rohdewald has overseen safety studies of Pycnogenol since 1982. He is a pharmaceutical researcher and teaches pharmaceutical science. He is well versed in toxicology and the safety of nutrients and drugs and has served as the Commissarial Director of the Institute for Pharmaceutical Chemistry at the University of Muenster.

Several acute toxicity studies found that it would take 336 grams—nearly one pound—to cause any type of toxic effects in a 155-pound person. Studies of long-term toxicity found that adverse effects would not be produced until 35,000 milligrams a day were taken for more than six months by a 155-pound person. The highest recommended dose of Pycnogenol is about 155 milligrams a day for a 155-pound person, and more typical dosages would be in the 25 to 50 milligrams per day range. Pycnogenol is safe as a daily food supplement when taken as recommended.

Q. Who should take Pycnogenol?

A. There are no known contraindications—conditions under which Pycnogenol should not be used. Even pregnant women and small children can safely take advantage of the health benefits of Pycnogenol, although it is always wise for them to take any supplements or medication in moderation.

Conclusion

By now, you understand why Pycnogenol has excited so many people. It can help protect you from a variety of diseases—including various types of heart disease and circulatory disorders—aggravated by free radicals. It can boost your immune system and also help protect you from infectious diseases.

As scientists have become excited about Pycnogenol, it has motivated them to investigate and discover the specific and highly detailed mechanisms of how it works. They are learning about how Pycnogenol interacts with nitric oxide, cellular adhesion molecules, and many other other biochemical molecules.

Such details may not be of interest to you. Odds are that the health benefits of Pycnogenol are of much greater interest. In writing about Pycnogenol and in frequently talking with scientists doing the actual research on this remarkable substance, I have continued to be impressed by its positive effects on health. Obviously, I take it myself, and, perhaps not surprisingly, I think that everyone could benefit from Pycnogenol supplements.

Glossary

Aggregation. Assembling, clumping, or sticking together.

Antioxidant. Compounds that protect other compounds against oxidation and free radicals.

Bioavailability. The rate at which a nutrient is made available for action in the body.

Bioflavonoids. A family of beneficial compounds with a crystalline structure, which are found in plants.

Collagen. A protein that composes much of connective tissue and skin.

Enzymes. Proteins that initiate specific reactions in the body.

Free radical. An atom or molecule with at least one unpaired electron that damages body components and can lead to many diseases.

Oxidation. The reaction of a compound with oxygen, or a reaction in which an atom loses an electron.

Platelets. Small blood cells involved in forming blood clots.

Proanthocyanidins. Another name for procyanidins.

Procyanidins. A subclass of bioflavonoids to which Pycnogenol belongs.

Pycnogenol. A nutritional supplement, composed of bioflavonoids and organic acids, that has several beneficial effects in the body, including antioxidant activities, immune boosting effects, and cardiovascular protective properties.

References

Blazso, G, et al., "Antiinflammatory and super-oxide radical scavenging activities of a pro-cyanidins-containing extract from the bark of *Pinus pinaster Sol.* and its fractions," *Pharm Pharmacol Letters* 3(1994): 217–230.

Cheshier, JE, et al, "Immunomodulation by Pycnogenol in retrovirus-infected or ethanol-fed mice," *Life Sci.* 58 (1996): 87–96.

Guochang, A, "Ultraviolet radiation-induced oxidative stress in cultured human skin fibrob-lasts and antioxidant protection," *Biological Research Reports from the University of Jyvaskla* 33 (1993): 1–86.

Passwater, Richard A, "Pycnogenol Research Update: An interview with Dr. Peter Rohdewald," *Whole Foods* (August 1997): 46–49.

Rohdewald, P, "Pycnogenol" in *Flavonoids in Health and Disease*, Evans and Packer, eds., NY: Marcel Dekker, Inc., 1997.

Rong, Y, et al., "Pycnogenol protects vascular endothelial cells from t-butyl hydroperoxide," *Biotech Ther* 95(5) (1994):117–126.

Tixier, JM, et al., "Evidence by *in vivo* and *in vitro* studies that binding of pycnogenols to elastin affects its rate of degradation by elastases," *Biochem. Pharmacol.* 33 (1984): 3933–3939.

Virgili, F, et al., "Nitrogen monoxide metabolism" in *Flavonoids in Health and Disease*, Evans and Packer, eds., NY: Marcel Dekker, Inc., 1997.

Suggested Readings

Passwater, Richard A. *The New Superantioxidant—Plus*. New Canaan, CT: Keats Publishing, 1992.

Passwater, Richard A. *Pycnogenol: The Super "Protector" Nutrient*. New Canaan, CT: Keats Publishing, 1994.

Index